Easy Weight Loss Plans

Best ways to loss 10 pounds without lifting weight

Warren .A. Richardson

Table of Contents

Introduction: Easy Weight Loss Plans

Welcome to "Easy Weight Loss Plans: A Holistic Approach to Weight Loss and Well-Being without lifting Weights." This eBook is your comprehensive guide to achieving your weight loss goals while embracing a holistic and sustainable approach to health and wellness. Within these pages, you'll embark on a journey that goes beyond simply shedding pounds; you'll discover how to nourish your body, nurture your mind, and cultivate a vibrant, balanced life.

In a world filled with fad diets and quick fixes, we believe in the power of a holistic approach—one that considers your physical, mental, and emotional well-being. True transformation involves more than just changing what you eat; it consists in shifting your mindset, embracing mindful habits, fostering a supportive community, and creating a lifestyle that supports your long-term goals.

This eBook is designed to be your companion on this journey, offering you a roadmap to navigate the challenges and triumphs that come with pursuing a healthier lifestyle. Each chapter explores a different facet of your journey, from understanding the foundations of weight loss to mastering mindful eating, from harnessing the power of superfoods to enjoying dining out without derailing your progress.

As you read through these pages, take time to reflect on how each concept resonates with you. Consider how you can integrate these insights into your daily life, transforming them into practical, sustainable habits. Remember that this journey is uniquely yours, and every step you take is a testament to your dedication and resilience.

Whether you're just beginning your weight loss journey or seeking to enhance your existing approach, "Easy Weight Loss Plans" is here to guide you every step of the way. Get ready to embark on a transformation that encompasses not only your physical body but also your mind, spirit, and overall well-being. Your empowered journey starts now.

Let's dive in!

Chapter 1: The Foundation of Weight Loss

Welcome to the first chapter of your transformative journey toward a healthier, more vibrant you! As you embark on this adventure, we'll explore the essential elements that lay the groundwork for successful weight loss—starting with the cornerstone of it all: The Foundation of a Healthy Diet.

Healthy Diet: Unveiling the Power of Balanced Nutrition

Imagine your body as a complex, high-performance machine—one that requires the finest fuel to operate at its peak. This is where a balanced diet steps in, acting as the fuel that not only energizes your body but also fuels your weight loss journey.

Lean Proteins: Just as a sturdy frame supports a building, lean proteins are the building blocks that support your body's growth, repair, and overall functionality. Think of lean proteins as your body's construction workers, repairing

Tissues and building lean muscle mass. Opt for sources like chicken, turkey, fish, beans, and tofu to keep your protein intake well-balanced.

Whole Grains: Picture whole grains as the solid foundation upon which your diet rests. These grains provide sustained energy, essential nutrients, and dietary fiber that aids in digestion and satiety. Whole grains like quinoa, brown rice, whole wheat, and oats should take center stage in your diet, replacing refined grains that can lead to energy crashes and overeating.

Vibrant Fruits and Nourishing Vegetables: Imagine a palette of vibrant colors painted on your plate. This is where fruits and vegetables come in, delivering an array of vitamins, minerals, and antioxidants that bolster your body's defense mechanisms. From the antioxidant-rich blues of blueberries to the vibrant orange of carrots, these foods not only nourish but also add a delightful burst of flavor to your meals.

Portion Control: The Art of Mindful Consumption

Now that you have the ingredients for a balanced diet, let's explore how to serve those ingredients in just the right proportions. Imagine portion control as the conductor of a symphony—balancing different elements to create a harmonious masterpiece.

Caloric Management: Visualize your body as a scale that needs to maintain equilibrium. Consuming too many calories tilts the scale towards weight gain while consuming too few calories can lead to deprivation and slow metabolism.

Portion control ensures you're striking the perfect balance, helping you lose weight while still enjoying satisfying meals.

Mindful Eating: Imagine savoring every bite of your meal, fully immersed in the sensory experience. Mindful eating encourages you to slow down, engage your senses, and recognize when you're genuinely satisfied. This practice empowers you to honor your body's hunger cues and avoid the common pitfall of overeating.

Tricks to Train Your Brain: Consider your brain as the conductor of your body's orchestra, shaping your eating habits and responses. By using smaller plates, bowls, and utensils, you can trick your brain into perceiving larger portions, leading you to feel more satisfied with less food. Moreover, focusing on each bite and taking breaks during your meal can help your brain catch up with your stomach, preventing overindulgence.

Regular Meals: The Rhythm of Sustained Energy

Imagine your body as a finely tuned instrument that thrives on consistency and rhythm. Regular, balanced meals and snacks serve as the metronome, ensuring your energy levels remain steady throughout the day.

Stabilizing Blood Sugar: Visualize your body's energy levels as a roller coaster. Skipping meals or waiting too long between meals can send your energy plummeting, leading to ravenous overeating later on. Regular meals and snacks maintain stable blood sugar levels, preventing energy crashes and keeping those unhealthy cravings at bay.

Optimizing Metabolism: Picture your metabolism as a blazing fire that requires a constant supply of fuel. By spacing out your meals and eating at regular intervals, you stoke your metabolic fire, encouraging efficient calorie burning and weight loss.

Strategic Meal Timing: Imagine your meals as carefully choreographed dance routines. Eating a balanced breakfast jumpstarts your metabolism, while spaced-out meals and a satisfying dinner nourish your body throughout the day. This strategic approach prevents nighttime binging and allows your body to burn calories efficiently.

As you conclude this chapter, reflect on the powerful role a healthy diet, portion control, and regular meals play in laying the foundation for your weight loss journey. Your journey is not about deprivation but rather about embracing the delightful world of balanced nutrition, mindful eating, and strategic meal timing. Armed with this knowledge, you're ready to take the next steps toward achieving your weight loss goals, transforming your body, and ultimately, your life.

Chapter 2: Lifestyle Factors for Success

Welcome to Chapter 2 of your empowering journey toward achieving your weight loss goals! In this chapter, we'll delve into the lifestyle factors that serve as the compass guiding you toward success—beyond the confines of a traditional gym setting.

Hydration: Nourishing Your Body's Oasis

Imagine your body as a lush oasis in the midst of a desert, with hydration acting as the lifeblood that sustains your vitality and progress.

Water's Vital Role: Visualize water as the foundation upon which your body's functions are built. Adequate hydration supports digestion, circulation, temperature regulation, and even the transportation of nutrients. By drinking enough water, you ensure your body functions optimally, enhancing your weight loss journey.

Thirst vs. Hunger: Picture thirst and hunger as two travelers in the same desert. Often, your body confuses thirst for hunger, leading you to eat unnecessarily. By staying hydrated, you can differentiate between these signals, preventing overeating and keeping your calorie intake in check.

Hydration and Skin Health: Imagine hydration as the elixir of glowing skin. Well-hydrated skin appears plump and vibrant, a visual testament to your body's well-being. Drinking water supports healthy skin, promoting a radiant appearance as you progress on your journey.

Mindful Eating: Savoring Every Sensation

Now, let's delve into the concept of mindful eating—a practice that encourages you to be fully present during meals, savoring every bite and sensation.

Eating with Awareness: Imagine your meals as a captivating performance. Mindful eating encourages you to put away distractions and focus solely on your meal, allowing you to appreciate flavors, textures, and aromas. This practice not only enhances your eating experience but also helps prevent overeating.

Listening to Your Body: Visualize your body as a wise friend who communicates its needs through subtle cues. Mindful eating teaches you to tune in to these cues, recognizing when you're truly hungry and when you're satisfied. By understanding your body's signals, you gain better control over your eating habits.

Preventing Emotional Eating: Picture emotions as waves that can sometimes engulf your better judgment. Mindful eating equips you with the tools to identify emotional triggers for eating and develop healthier ways to cope with stress, sadness, or boredom. This practice fosters a balanced relationship with food, untethered from emotional impulses.

Physical Activity: Unveiling the Joy of Movement

Imagine your body as a vessel designed for movement, ready to explore a myriad of physical activities that contribute to your weight loss journey.

Beyond the Gym: Visualize physical activity not as a confined space but as a vast playground encompassing various enjoyable pursuits. Engage in activities like walking, dancing, gardening, and recreational sports—these contribute to calorie burning and improved cardiovascular health without the pressure of traditional gym workouts.

The Joy of Exploration: Picture your body as an adventurer eager to discover new horizons. By experimenting with different activities, you'll find forms of movement that resonate with you, transforming exercise from a chore to a delightful pastime.

Consistency Over Intensity: Imagine consistency as the cornerstone of successful physical activity. Regular movement, even in small increments, accumulates over time and supports your weight loss efforts. Strive for sustainability, making physical activity an integral part of your lifestyle.

As you conclude this chapter, reflect on the profound impact that hydration, mindful eating, and physical activity have on your weight loss journey. These lifestyle factors go beyond the traditional approach, allowing you to find joy, balance, and fulfillment on your path to a healthier you. With each step, you're building a strong foundation for lifelong success—one that prioritizes self-care, mindfulness, and the enjoyment of movement.

Chapter 3: Holistic Health Approach

Welcome to Chapter 3, where we delve into the holistic aspects of your weight loss journey. Here, we'll explore how sleep, stress management, and healthy snacking play pivotal roles in achieving your goals.

Sleep: Nurturing Your Body's Sanctuary

Imagine sleep as a sacred sanctuary, where your body rejuvenates, repairs, and prepares for the challenges of each day.

Quality Over Quantity: Visualize sleep as a treasure chest of rejuvenation. Prioritize both the duration and quality of your sleep to ensure your body's internal systems function optimally. Adequate sleep fosters hormone regulation, supporting your weight loss efforts.

Hormones and Hunger: Picture hormones as conductors of your body's orchestra. Sleep deprivation disrupts the harmony of these hormones, leading to increased appetite and cravings for high-calorie foods. By prioritizing sleep, you regain control over your hunger cues.

Energy and Focus: Imagine sleep as a wellspring of energy that fuels your activities and decision-making. A well-rested body is better equipped to engage in physical activity, make healthier food choices, and resist impulsive snacking.

Stress Management: Navigating Life's Waters

Now, let's explore stress management—an essential skill that empowers you to navigate life's challenges without resorting to emotional eating.

Understanding Stress: Visualize stress as turbulent waters that can throw your weight loss journey off course. Stress triggers the release of cortisol, a hormone that promotes fat storage, particularly in the abdominal region. By managing stress, you prevent unnecessary weight gain.

Mind-Body Techniques: Picture stress management techniques as life vests, keeping you afloat during challenging times. Practices such as meditation, deep breathing, and mindfulness cultivate a sense of calm, helping you avoid stress-induced overeating.

Embracing Resilience: Imagine resilience as a protective shield that guards against emotional eating. Through stress management techniques, you build resilience, allowing you to cope with stressors in healthier ways and maintain your commitment to a balanced diet.

Healthy Snacking: Nourishing Your In-Between Moments

Now, let's explore the world of healthy snacking—a practice that ensures you stay nourished and satisfied throughout the day.

Smart Snacking Choices: Visualize healthy snacks as miniature nutrient powerhouses. Opt for snacks like nuts, yogurt, fruits, and vegetables, which provide essential vitamins, minerals, and fiber without excess calories.

Preventing Overindulgence: Picture healthy snacks as checkpoints that prevent overeating during main meals. By incorporating balanced snacks between meals, you avoid arriving at your next meal with intense hunger, which can lead to overconsumption.

Mindful Snacking: Imagine mindful snacking as a delightful ritual. Engage your senses while enjoying your snack, savoring each bite and practicing portion control. This mindfulness fosters a healthy relationship with food, eliminating guilt associated with indulgence.

As you conclude this chapter, reflect on the profound impact that sleep, stress management, and healthy snacking have on your holistic health journey. By prioritizing sleep, managing stress effectively, and making mindful choices when snacking, you're nurturing your body's well-being from multiple angles. Your journey is not just about weight loss—it's about cultivating a harmonious connection between your physical, mental, and emotional aspects. With these holistic practices in your toolkit, you're poised to navigate challenges with resilience and relish in the joys of a balanced, health-focused lifestyle.

Chapter 4: Mindset Shifts for Success

Welcome to Chapter 4, a realm where we dive into the psychology of your weight loss journey. Here, we explore the power of your mindset, uncovering techniques that will empower you to achieve your goals.

The Psychology of Weight Loss

Imagine your mindset as the compass that directs your actions. A positive mindset can be your greatest ally, guiding you toward success with every step.

Self-Compassion: Visualize self-compassion as a warm embrace you extend to yourself. Instead of berating yourself for slip-ups, cultivate kindness. Treat yourself as you would a dear friend, acknowledging that setbacks are part of the journey.

Setting Realistic Goals: Picture goals as stepping stones toward your destination. By setting achievable goals, you avoid the pitfalls of frustration and disappointment. Each small victory adds up, leading you closer to your ultimate success.

Positive Visualization: Imagine success as a vivid image in your mind's eye. Visualize yourself achieving your weight loss goals, feeling the emotions of accomplishment and pride. This mental rehearsal empowers you to manifest your aspirations.

Identifying Triggers: Visualize self-sabotage triggers as warning signs on the road ahead. Recognize situations, emotions, or habits that lead to unhealthy choices. Awareness empowers you to make conscious decisions.

Replacing Negative Habits: Picture habits as well-worn paths in your mind. Replace negative habits with positive alternatives. For instance, if stress triggers emotional eating, explore stress-relief techniques instead.

Embracing Flexibility: Imagine flexibility as a safety net. Life is filled with unexpected twists, and setbacks are normal. Instead of derailing your progress, approach setbacks as opportunities to learn and adjust your course.

Goal Setting and Celebrating Progress

Now, let's delve into effective goal setting and celebrating your progress—two practices that fuel your motivation.

SMART Goals: Visualize SMART goals as roadmaps to success. Make your goals Specific, Measurable, Achievable, Relevant, and Time-bound. This framework provides clarity and direction, making your journey manageable.

Progress Tracking: Imagine progress tracking as a GPS guiding you. Regularly monitor your achievements, recording your weight, measurements, or fitness milestones. This data-driven approach highlights your progress, motivating you to continue.

Non-Scale Victories: Picture victories beyond the scale. Celebrate improved energy levels, better sleep, increased strength, or fitting into clothing better. These non-scale triumphs reinforce your commitment to a healthier lifestyle.

As you conclude this chapter, reflect on the power of your mindset and the strategies that empower you to overcome self-sabotage. With a positive mindset, you're equipped to tackle challenges with resilience and embrace the journey's transformative nature. By setting realistic goals, replacing negative habits, and celebrating progress, you're actively shaping your path to success. The journey is not just about physical transformation—it's about nurturing your inner world and paving the way for lasting change. With the right mindset, you're unstoppable in your quest to achieve your weight loss goals.

Chapter 5: Nutrient-Rich Superfoods

Welcome to Chapter 5, where we dive into the vibrant world of nutrient-rich superfoods. In this chapter, we'll explore a cornucopia of foods that can turbocharge your weight loss journey with their powerhouse nutrients.

Superfoods: Nature's Nutrient Powerhouses

Imagine super foods as nature's secret weapons, brimming with an array of vitamins, minerals, antioxidants, and other essential compounds that fuel your body's transformation.

Kale: Picture kale as a leafy green superhero, bursting with vitamins A, C, and K. It's also a source of fiber, iron, and antioxidants that support your overall health.

Berries: Imagine berries as antioxidant-rich gems that add a burst of flavor and color to your meals. Blueberries, strawberries, and raspberries offer a potent dose of vitamins and phytonutrients.

Incorporating Superfoods into Your Diet

Now, let's explore how to incorporate these superfoods into your meals and snacks, enhancing your nutrient intake and accelerating your weight loss progress.

Smoothie Boosters: Visualize super foods as the secret ingredients that transform your smoothies into nutrient powerhouses. Add chia seeds, berries, and a handful of kale to your smoothie for an energizing start to your day.

Salad Stars: Picture Super Foods as the star players in your salads. Create colorful salads with a base of nutrient-rich kale, topped with berries, nuts, and seeds for added texture and flavor.

Chia Puddings: Imagine chia seeds as the magic behind creamy chia puddings. Mix chia seeds with your favorite milk and let them soak to create a satisfying and nutrient-dense snack.

Super Foods for Sustained Success

Now, let's explore how superfoods contribute to your sustained success on your weight loss journey.

Satiety and Satisfaction: Visualize super foods as allies in curbing cravings and promoting satiety. Their nutrient density helps you feel satisfied, reducing the likelihood of overeating.

Energy and Vitality: Picture superfoods as a natural energy boost. The vitamins, minerals, and antioxidants they provide support your body's energy production, keeping you vibrant and active.

Long-Term Health: Imagine superfoods as an investment in your long-term health. The compounds they contain help protect against chronic diseases, promoting overall wellness beyond weight loss.

As you conclude this chapter, reflect on the abundance of nutrient-rich superfoods that can elevate your weight loss journey. By incorporating these foods into your diet, you're providing your body with the essential nutrients it craves, accelerating your progress, and nurturing your health from the inside out. Embrace the variety and flavors that superfoods bring to your meals, and savor the knowledge that you're fueling your transformation with nature's finest offerings.

Chapter 6: Meal Prep Mastery

Welcome to Chapter 6, a culinary adventure that will empower you to master the art of meal prepping. In this chapter, we'll explore the world of organized meal planning and preparation—a strategy that can streamline your weight loss journey and set you up for success.

The Magic of Meal Prep

Imagine meal prep as a magical ritual that transforms your week ahead. This practice involves planning, preparing, and packaging your meals in advance, saving you time, reducing stress, and supporting your weight loss goals.

Efficiency and Convenience: Visualize meal prep as a time-saving treasure trove. Spending dedicated time on meal prep ensures that healthy, balanced meals are ready whenever you need them, minimizing last-minute decisions and potential indulgences.

Portion Control: Picture meal prep as your ally in portion control. By pre-portioning your meals, you eliminate the guesswork and reduce the likelihood of overeating.

Variety and Flavor: Imagine meal prep as an opportunity to explore diverse cuisines and flavors. Prepare a range of dishes using lean proteins, whole grains, and vibrant vegetables to keep your taste buds excited.

Mastering the Art of Meal Prep

Now, let's dive into practical steps to become a meal prep maestro, ensuring that your efforts translate into a seamless and enjoyable experience.

Planning Ahead: Visualize meal planning as the blueprint of your culinary journey. Set aside time to plan your meals for the week, considering your schedule, dietary preferences, and nutritional needs.

Batch Cooking: Picture batch cooking as the backbone of meal prep. Prepare larger quantities of staple ingredients like grains, proteins, and vegetables, making it easy to assemble meals throughout the week.

Smart Storage: Imagine meal storage as the final touch to your culinary creations. Invest in quality storage containers to keep your meals fresh and organized. Choose transparent containers to admire the colorful layers of your dishes.

The Benefits of Meal Prep

Now, let's explore the numerous benefits of meal prepping that extend beyond weight loss.

Nutritional Consistency: Visualize meal prep as a tool for nutritional consistency. When you control the ingredients and portions, you're more likely to adhere to your weight loss plan, supporting your progress.

Financial Savings: Picture meal prep as a wise financial investment. By planning your meals and shopping strategically, you minimize food waste and potentially save money.

Stress Reduction: Imagine meal prep as a stress-relief strategy. Having pre-made meals on hand eliminates the pressure of deciding what to eat during busy days, reducing stress and supporting mindful eating.

As you conclude this chapter, reflect on the transformative power of meal prepping. By planning, preparing, and packaging your meals, you're creating a roadmap for success—a journey where balanced nutrition, portion control, and convenience converge. Embrace meal prep as a gift you give yourself, simplifying your life and setting the stage for a triumphant weight loss journey.

Chapter 7: Social Support Networks

Welcome to Chapter 7, where we explore the invaluable role that social connections play in your weight loss journey. In this chapter, we'll delve into the power of community, whether through friends, family, or online networks, to provide motivation, accountability, and the sense of belonging that propels you forward.

The Strength of Community

Imagine your weight loss journey as a grand expedition, and your support network as fellow adventurers who walk alongside you, share experiences, and provide guidance.

Motivation and Encouragement: Visualize your support network as a wellspring of motivation. Connecting with others who share your goals creates a dynamic environment where accomplishments are celebrated, and challenges are met with encouragement.

Accountability: Picture accountability as the compass that keeps you on track. Sharing your goals and progress with others creates a sense of responsibility, encouraging you to stick to your commitments and maintain your momentum.

Empathy and Understanding: Imagine your support network as a refuge of empathy. They understand the highs and lows of the journey, providing a safe space where you can share your struggles and triumphs without judgment.

Building Your Support Network

Now, let's explore how to cultivate and nurture your support network, ensuring that it becomes a cornerstone of your weight loss success.

Family and Friends: Visualize your family and friends as your first circle of support. Share your goals and aspirations with loved ones, inviting them to join your journey and provide encouragement.

Online Communities: Picture online communities as virtual meeting places where like-minded individuals gather to exchange experiences and advice. Platforms and forums focused on health and wellness can be excellent sources of motivation and information.

Accountability Partners: Imagine accountability partners as fellow travelers on the same path. Pair up with someone who shares your goals, committing to support each other, celebrate achievements, and offer guidance during challenges.

The Power of Connection

Now, let's explore the remarkable impact that social connections can have on your well-being beyond weight loss.

Reduced Stress: Visualize your support network as a cushion against stress. Engaging with others who understand your journey provides an outlet to discuss challenges, share coping strategies, and receive reassurance.

Enhanced Motivation: Picture your support network as a chorus of cheerleaders. When you see others achieving their goals and making progress, you're inspired to stay committed and continue your efforts.

Long-Term Benefits: Imagine your support network as a lifelong asset. As you cultivate these connections, you're not only supporting your current weight loss journey but also creating a network that can help you maintain a healthy lifestyle in the years to come.

As you conclude this chapter, reflect on the potential of your social support network to elevate your weight loss journey. By engaging with a community that shares your aspirations, you're creating a dynamic ecosystem of motivation, accountability, and shared experiences. Embrace the connections that come your way, for they have the power to uplift, inspire, and propel you toward your goals like never before.

Chapter 8: Enjoying Dining Out

Welcome to Chapter 8, where we navigate the delightful world of dining out without compromising your weight loss goals. In this chapter, we'll explore strategies to make informed choices, manage portion sizes, and savor the experience of eating out while staying true to your journey.

The Art of Mindful Dining

Imagine dining out as an opportunity to savor not only the flavors of the cuisine but also the joy of socializing and indulging in a delightful experience.

Preparation: Visualize preparation as your dining out compass. Before heading to a restaurant, explore the menu online and choose dishes that align with your goals and preferences.

Portion Control: Picture portion control as the key to dining out success. Many restaurants serve larger portions than you may need. Consider sharing dishes, ordering appetizers as main courses, or asking for a to-go container to pack leftovers.

Balanced Choices: Imagine balanced choices as the cornerstone of mindful dining. Opt for dishes that include lean proteins, vegetables, and whole grains. Request dressings and sauces on the side to control the amount you consume.

Navigating Different Cuisines

Now, let's explore how to navigate different types of cuisine, ensuring that your dining out experiences are diverse, enjoyable, and aligned with your goals.

Asian Cuisine: Visualize Asian cuisine as a tapestry of flavors and options. Choose dishes with lean proteins, vegetables, and minimal sauces. Avoid deep-fried items and opt for stir-fries or steamed dishes.

Italian Cuisine: Picture Italian cuisine as a celebration of simplicity. Opt for dishes that feature tomato-based sauces, grilled proteins, and whole-grain pasta. Limit creamy sauces and heavy cheeses.

Mexican Cuisine: Imagine Mexican cuisine as a colorful fiesta of flavors. Choose dishes with grilled proteins, vegetables, and salsa. Limit high-calorie extras like sour cream and opt for corn tortillas over flour tortillas.

Mindful Indulgence

Now, let's explore the art of mindful indulgence—an important aspect of dining out that allows you to enjoy treats while maintaining balance.

Savoring Treats: Visualize treats as occasional indulgences to be savored mindfully. Instead of feeling guilty, embrace the experience and enjoy a small portion of your favorite dessert or indulgent dish.

Compensating with Choices: Picture compensating as a way to balance indulgence. If you plan to enjoy a richer dish, make healthier choices throughout the day or increase your physical activity to maintain your overall calorie balance.

Finding Satisfaction: Imagine satisfaction as the heart of mindful indulgence. Enjoy your treat fully, paying attention to each bite and truly relishing the experience. This approach prevents feelings of deprivation and overindulgence.

As you conclude this chapter, reflect on the strategies that allow you to enjoy dining out while staying aligned with your weight loss journey. By approaching dining out with mindfulness, preparation, and balanced choices, you're transforming restaurant visits into enjoyable, guilt-free experiences. Embrace the variety of cuisines and flavors the world offers, and remember that dining out can be an enriching part of your journey—one that nourishes both your body and your spirit.

Chapter 9: Sustainable Habits for Life

Welcome to Chapter 9, the culmination of your journey towards achieving your weight loss goals. In this chapter, we'll explore how to transition from a focused weight loss phase to a sustainable lifestyle that nurtures your health, well-being, and lasting success.

The Journey Continues

Imagine your weight loss journey as a river flowing into the vast ocean of your life. As you reach your goals, the journey doesn't end—it transforms into a sustainable way of living.

Lifestyle Shifts: Visualize lifestyle shifts as the natural progression of your journey. Embrace the habits you've cultivated along the way, from balanced nutrition and portion control to mindful eating and regular physical activity.

Long-Term Vision: Picture your journey as a tapestry woven with long-term aspirations. Shift your focus from short-term goals to maintaining your progress and cultivating a vibrant, healthy life.

Enjoying Balance: Imagine balance as the heart of sustainability. Continue to enjoy the foods you love while making mindful choices. Balance indulgences with nutrient-dense meals and find joy in both.

Cultivating Holistic Wellness

Now, let's explore how your journey extends beyond weight loss to encompass holistic wellness—nurturing your mind, body, and spirit.

Self-Care Rituals: Visualize self-care as the cornerstone of your well-being. Engage in activities that bring you joy, reduce stress, and promote relaxation, whether it's reading, practicing yoga, or spending time in nature.

Mind-Body Connection: Picture the mind-body connection as a bridge between your thoughts and your physical well-being. Cultivate mindfulness through meditation, deep breathing, and gratitude to enhance your overall quality of life.

Staying Active: Imagine staying active as a lifelong commitment. Choose physical activities you enjoy, whether it's dancing, hiking, or practicing a sport. Consistent movement contributes to your energy, vitality, and longevity.

Embracing the Journey

Now, let's explore the essence of embracing your journey as a continuous evolution, a tapestry of experiences that shape your growth.

Reflection and Progress: Visualize reflection as a way to celebrate how far you've come. Regularly review your achievements, revisit your goals, and acknowledge the positive changes you've made.

Flexibility and Adaptability: Picture flexibility as your companion on this journey. Life is filled with changes, and your approach may need to adapt. Embrace flexibility, knowing that setbacks are temporary and adjustments are part of progress.

Reaching Out: Imagine reaching out as an acknowledgment of your growth. Share your experiences and insights with others, supporting those who embark on similar journeys and contributing to a community of wellness.

As you conclude this chapter, reflect on the transformation you've undergone and the sustainable habits you've cultivated. Your journey isn't confined to a single phase—it's a lifelong commitment to nurturing your health, well-being, and happiness. Embrace each day with a sense of purpose and gratitude, knowing that your journey is a testament to your resilience, dedication, and the incredible potential within you.

Chapter 10: Your Journey Ahead

Welcome to Chapter 10, the final chapter of this eBook. In this chapter, we'll take a moment to reflect on your journey, celebrate your achievements, and provide you with a roadmap for continued success and growth.

Reflecting on Your Transformation

Imagine this moment as a pause in your journey, a chance to reflect on how far you've come since the beginning.

Celebrating Achievements: Visualize a gallery of your accomplishments. Celebrate not only your weight loss milestones but also the new habits, insights, and mindset shift you've embraced along the way.

Inner Transformation: Picture your journey as a tapestry of inner change. Reflect on how your relationship with food, your body, and your self-esteem has evolved, setting the stage for a happier, healthier you.

Life beyond Weight: Imagine your journey expanding beyond weight loss. Your newfound vitality and confidence influence various aspects of your life—your relationships, work, hobbies, and the way you engage with the world.

Navigating the Future

Now, let's explore how to navigate the exciting path ahead, armed with the tools and wisdom you've gained.

Setting New Goals: Visualize setting new goals as a compass guiding you forward. Whether it's building on your fitness, exploring a new activity, or deepening your self-care routine, continue to challenge and inspire yourself.

Maintaining Balance: Picture balance as the key to lasting success. Embrace a lifestyle that integrates nutritious eating, enjoyable physical activities, and mindful practices, ensuring you enjoy every facet of your life.

Staying Connected: Imagine staying connected as a way to nurture your growth. Continue engaging with your support network, sharing your experiences, and learning from others. This community remains a source of encouragement and insight.

Embracing the Journey

Now, let's explore the essence of embracing the journey—an ongoing adventure filled with growth, self-discovery, and endless possibilities.

Gratitude: Visualize gratitude as the foundation of your journey. Embrace each step with appreciation, acknowledging the challenges, the triumphs, and the lessons they bring.

Inspiring Others: Picture your journey as an inspiration to those around you. By sharing your story and the strategies you've learned, you contribute to a ripple effect of positive change in the lives of others.

Continual Evolution: Imagine your journey as a river that flows with the currents of change. Embrace the evolution of your goals, your strategies, and yourself, knowing that growth is a constant companion.

As you conclude this eBook, take a moment to absorb the wisdom and insights you've gained throughout these chapters. You've embarked on a transformative journey—one that goes beyond weight loss to encompass holistic well-being, mindset shifts, and sustainable habits. Embrace the path ahead with excitement, knowing that you are equipped with the knowledge, tools, and support to create a life of vitality, balance, and joy. Your journey is a testament to your resilience, dedication, and the incredible potential within you. Embrace each day as a new opportunity to thrive and continue on the extraordinary journey you've embarked upon.

Conclusion: Your Empowered Journey

Congratulations on reaching the conclusion of this eBook! Your journey towards achieving your weight loss goals has been a remarkable adventure filled with discovery, growth, and transformation. As you stand at this juncture, take a moment to acknowledge the strides you've made and the positive changes you've embraced.

Remember that your journey is not just about shedding pounds—it's about cultivating a vibrant, balanced life that nourishes your body, mind, and spirit. The chapters in this eBook have guided you through a holistic approach to weight loss, offering insights into healthy eating, mindful habits, lifestyle adjustments, and the power of community.

As you move forward, carry these key takeaways with you:

Holistic Health: Embrace the interconnectedness of your physical, mental, and emotional well-being. Your journey is not just about the numbers on the scale—it's about nurturing every facet of your being.

Mindset Matters: Your mindset is the compass that guides your actions. Cultivate a positive, resilient mindset that empowers you to overcome challenges and stay committed to your goals.

Sustainable Habits: Focus on building sustainable habits that will serve you for a lifetime. It's not just about reaching your destination—it's about creating a lifestyle that supports your well-being.

Community and Support: Surround yourself with a supportive network of friends, family, and like-minded individuals. These connections provide motivation, encouragement, and a sense of belonging.

Enjoy the Journey: Your journey is a process of growth and self-discovery. Embrace each step with gratitude and enthusiasm, knowing that every choice you make contributes to your progress.

As you move forward, remember that your journey is uniquely yours. It's filled with ups and downs, twists and turns, but it's also rich with opportunities for growth and transformation. Your potential is limitless, and your commitment to your well-being is a testament to your strength and determination.

Thank you for embarking on this journey with us. Your dedication to creating a healthier, happier you is truly inspiring. Embrace the future with confidence, knowing that you have the tools, knowledge, and resilience to achieve your goals and live a life that radiates vitality, balance, and joy. Your empowered journey continues, and the possibilities are endless.